The TROOTH in DENTISTRY

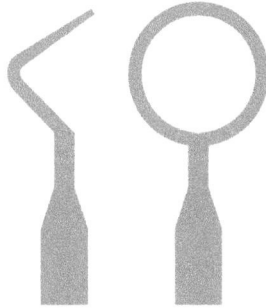

Ryan C. Maher, DMD

For more information contact:
Dr. Ryan C. Maher, DMD
drryanmaher@gmail.com
http://www.thetroothindentistry.com/

978-0-692-41328-9 hard cover
978-0-692-41329-6 ebook

Library of Congress Control Number: 2014916922

CONTENTS

CHAPTER 1

Needles and X-rays and Drills, Oh My!

RIGHT NOW, SOMEWHERE in the United States, someone in a dentist's chair is in pain—not the kind of pain associated with oral infection or disease, but the kind of pain that comes from receiving improper care. The sound of the drill is thrumming through every bone in his skull. He can smell the tips of his oral nerve endings being torched. Though his eyes are shut tight in an effort to keep the tears from streaming down his face, he knows his gloved and masked torturer is hovering over him, mere inches from his propped-open mouth. These

> Right now, somewhere in the United States, someone in a dentist's chair is in pain—not the kind of pain associated with oral infection or disease, but the kind of pain that comes from receiving improper care.

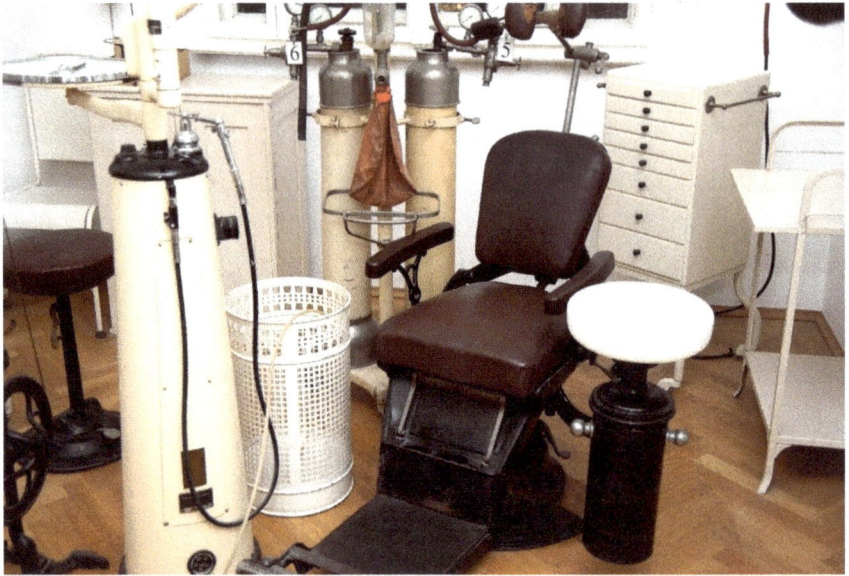

patients, experiencing this pain, feel absolute vulnerability. But the larger truth is that we are all this vulnerable when it comes to receiving the dental care we deserve.

Even if just one out of every ten patients reports experiencing pain during a dental visit, that is one patient too many. In the earliest days of professional dentistry—at around the time of the construction of the Egyptian pyramids—having a tooth pulled felt like … well, you can imagine! Five thousand years ago, the Chinese assigned some twenty-six acupuncture sites to toothache relief, and the Sumerians attributed all oral suffering to demons. Fast forward a few eras, and cocaine numbed the gums for dental procedures in North America throughout the nineteenth century. Novocaine made its debut in 1905. Think about the first electric dental drill—it was used in this country in 1870,[1] and it took

_____

1 http://www.istockphoto.com/photo/old-vintage-dentist-chair-14920822?st=05ee0

hours to complete just one filling. Think about all those root canals dentists performed starting in the 1830s.

The dental office has come a long way from these days!

We dentists know that stress hormones run high for a lot of our patients. People list all of the following fears factors when asked what comes to mind when they think about their next dental appointment: the needle, the

> Read these chapters thoroughly to learn all you need to know about basic oral care, what to look for in a dentist, and what kind of dentist deserves closer scrutiny.

pain, the drill, the invasiveness, the cost, lectures, bad memories, the sounds, the smells, complications, and poor service. All this anxiety is perfectly understandable, but this book is going to shed light on the final two (complications and poor service), in addition to offering an overall education on key points of oral health.

We've all seen and read about complications—and even deaths—from dental care gone horribly wrong. Could any of those have been prevented? If dentists followed better procedures and offered better service, patients would certainly experience less suffering.

Patients, this book is for you—read these chapters thoroughly to learn all you need to know about basic oral care, what to look for in a dentist, and what kind of dentist deserves closer scrutiny.

Of course, the science and art of dentistry are rapidly evolving. And contrary to popular belief, we dentists take no delight in the fear or "monster" mythology surrounding our profession. We embrace the development of drugs and other techniques to ease our patients' pain, and we rejoice as our tools and drills become faster and more efficient. Sterilization equipment and strict sanitation requirements are implemented to meet increased public health awareness and regulations. Laser technology, safer x-ray procedures, and the reclining dental chairs that some of our patients now fall asleep in have brought us a long way, and we hope to continue on that road. We hand out those free toothbrushes with our names on them not as a gimmick, but with the genuine hope that each and every one of our patients will pay stronger attention to good dental hygiene.

There is nothing more rewarding to your dentist than to see that you have been doing your job—taking care of your mouth—at home. Dentists are more aware than anyone of the value of a good smile. Putting aesthetics aside for a second, studies have shown that the health of your teeth and gums greatly affects your overall health and wellbeing. Poor dental hygiene can result in impaired eating and sleeping habits—you might eat less or choose softer foods, and you might be plagued by chronic pain. People with oral health concerns may avoid laughing and smiling out of embarrassment. They may avoid social contact, experience social isolation, and battle depression. Developing babies smile in the womb. Research has proven that people who smile more often live longer.

In an independent study conducted on behalf of the American Academy of Cosmetic Dentistry, 99.7 percent of Americans believe a smile is an important social asset. You might say, "Yes, but that's *cosmetic* dentistry; that's just about what people look like, and I don't care about those superficial judgments." But even if you don't die younger because you aren't big on smiling, or even if you smile a lot even though your teeth are in poor shape, there are other psychosocial issues you must face.

One study revealed that people are more likely to bail out on a second date with someone who has bad teeth than someone who lives with his or her parents. The same study showed that skill set and experience being equal, people with straight teeth are perceived to be 45 percent more employable than those with crooked teeth. Ron Gutman, CEO of HealthTap and TEDMED contributor, cites studies showing that people who smile are considered more likable, courteous, and competent. In addition, smiling reduces stress hormones and increases the production of mood-enhancing hormones. Think about it: smiling might help you in more ways than one during your next dental visit.

Of course, smiling at your dentist has not always come naturally—and that is understandable. Prior to cocaine and Novocaine, arsenic was used during dental procedures, and fillings contained mercury—as some still do now—but the mercury then did not bond to the silver, meaning it often leeched into the patient's bloodstream. Indeed, a bad tooth prior to the twentieth century could sometimes lead to death.

Dental schools provide their own interesting history of the dental profession. The first US dental school opened in Baltimore in 1840. Baltimore now hosts the National Museum of Dentistry, which prides itself on its "Smile Experience." Dentistry has come a long way since 1840, and teeth fascinate us now just as much as they fascinated ancient peoples who shaved and filed their bicuspids or encrusted them with turquoise, gold, and rubies. As noted, our teeth are as culturally important to us today as they were in the days when our very language was centered around them: something that irritates us sets our teeth on edge, we fight tooth and nail, and we escape by the skin of our teeth. The tooth fairy has her origin story in the ancient ritual of hiding a lost tooth so that nobody could steal it and use it to perform voodoo on you!

The following stories (straight from the news) may seem improbable, but unfortunately they are true:

PARENTS ACCUSE HAWAII DENTIST OF LEAVING DAUGHTER, 3, WITH BRAIN DAMAGE [2]

In 2014, a three-year-old Hawaii girl named Finley Boyle suffered massive brain damage after undergoing a dental procedure. A lawsuit filed against the dentist by the girl's parents alleged that improper medications with incorrect dosages had been administered to the girl.

2 http://www.cnn.com/2014/01/03/justice/hawaii-brain-damage-girl/index.html

MAN DIES AFTER WISDOM TEETH REMOVED[3]

In 2013, a twenty-four-year-old California man died unexpectedly after having his wisdom teeth removed. Marek Lapinski, a software developer from San Diego, experienced complications woke up coughing during the routine procedure and was given a powerful anesthetic known as propofol. Lapinski's condition deteriorated quickly, and he was brought to a hospital, where he died three days later. Subsequently his family and friends began to question the treatment he'd received from his oral surgeon. According to the hospital, paramedics said the surgeon had told them that Lapinski woke up and started coughing during the procedure, and was given propofol. CPR was started when Lapinski stopped breathing, and the paramedics were called. The paramedics reportedly found two pieces of surgical gauze in Lapinski's airway when they tried to intubate him...

3 http://abcnews.go.com/Health/man-dies-wisdom-teeth-removed/story?id=18869553

THREE GEORGIA BOYS DIE UNEXPECTEDLY AFTER DENTAL PROCEDURE[4]

And in 2011, three boys died suddenly in Atlanta, Georgia, after routine dental procedures. The three boys, aged 14 to 21, died within a month of one another, and all had their wisdom teeth extracted within one to three days before they died. One death was ruled to have been caused by a reaction to penicillin; the cause of death is not known in the other two cases, although bacterial infection was considered to be a possibility. An expert interviewed by ABC news said that infections are a leading cause of deaths during dental procedures, owing to the high concentration of bacteria in the human mouth. Other causes of death following dental procedures include reactions to anesthesia or inhalation of blood into the lungs.

---

4 http://www.cbs46.com/story/17793876/3-georiga-boys-die-unexpectedly-after-dental-proceedure

As if the dental profession doesn't already get enough bad PR from movies like *Marathon Man* and *The Dentist*, we now have to face these horrible true stories. As a community, we need to learn from these extremely unfortunate stories and band together to stop them from happening ever again.

So from now on, make your dental professional an ally, and visit your medical doctor at the very least once a year for a complete physical and thorough bloodwork. Always take your health very seriously and have any and all medical issues addressed and treated as necessary. Your dentist should be aware of all medications you are taking, including over-the-counter and herbal remedies, as well as vitamins. You should also disclose all medical conditions, past surgeries, allergies, and any bloodwork concerns. The more information your dentist has, the less chance for potential future problems.

> From now on, make your dental professional an ally, and visit your medical doctor at the very least once a year for a complete physical and thorough bloodwork.

This all begins with your medical history, so take your time filling it out. If your dentist is performing a surgical procedure, getting an okay from your MD might not be a bad idea, either. Let's also let time work in our favor, not against us, and not rush through dental procedures, especially surgical ones.

Rushing through a dental procedure can have several bad results. It sometimes happens that all the decay is not removed properly when a tooth is being prepared for a filling. I hate to say this, but I have found decay that was left in a tooth by another dentist after a standard dental procedure like a filling or a crown. Was the procedure rushed? Maybe. But regardless, decay is like a ticking time bomb in your mouth. If you pay a dentist $200 for a filling or two, and if that dentist leaves any decay, within a short time you may be in pain. And depending on the extent of the decay, your new dental bill could exceed $2,000.

Once the decay enters the nerve, a root canal is a must, and there is a high likelihood that a post and crown will be necessary as well. Yes, even when you are being the ideal dental patient—doing your job and taking good and timely care of your teeth—if a procedure is rushed, you may still pay the price.

Patients often cannot see what the dentist and his or her team should be able to see. Walking around with that time bomb of decay beneath the pretty surface of your stunning smile, you probably have no idea what you will soon be in for. If you have a crown that doesn't fit quite right, you may not feel anything is "off" when you bite down or when you chew your food, but even a slight gap in fit or size can result in food getting in where it isn't supposed to—which can lead to decay.

But how can you as a patient know about decay under a filling or recently done crown? It's not easy. Some indications may be that the crown comes out relatively soon, or that the filling breaks, or the tooth is getting food trapped where it never did in the past. A food trap is usually a red flag that something is wrong. When food gets trapped or stuck between teeth, it breaks down into bacteria that destroys the tooth.

With all that said, now is a good time to point out that dentistry is not the only field in which treatment fails or is sometimes not performed optimally. Search the Internet and I'm sure you will find countless medical mishaps—a doctor amputating the wrong leg, surgical instruments being left in the patient, and other fatal errors.

But this book is not meant to *increase* dental fears, nor is it meant to slander my peers. From a young age I knew I wanted to be a dentist, and I had the good fortune to know a great dentist who took the time to explain many of the wonders and basics of dentistry to me. From that exact point in my youth, I came to know—and still very much believe—that dentistry can be performed in an ethical, responsible, friendly, caring, and extremely precise manner.

At dental school, I learned to love the science and the art of the field, and eventually to understand the business of being a dentist. I wouldn't trade my job for any other. I am always thrilled to share information with my colleagues at conferences and in continuing education courses.

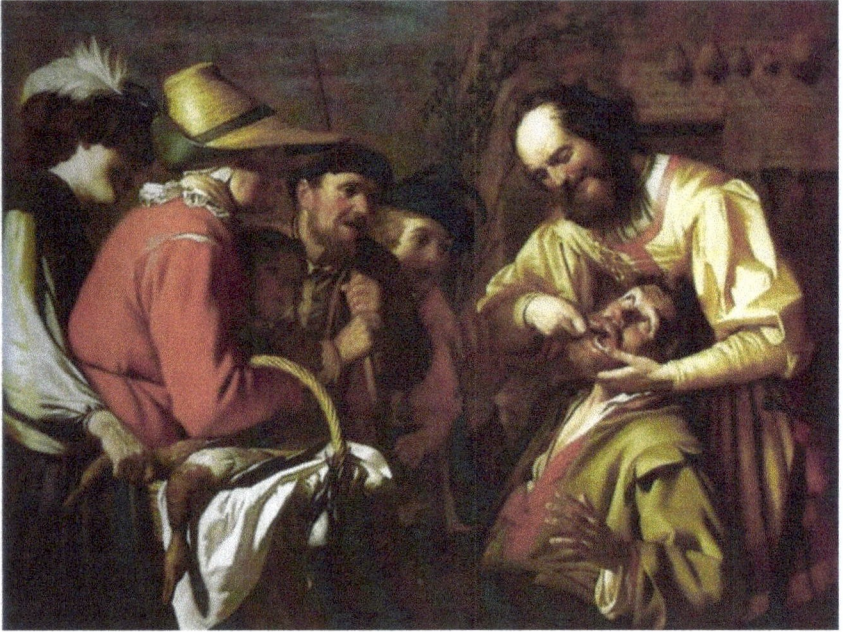

The Tooth Puller. Gerard van Honthorst. 1627.

This book is not meant to instill a fear bigger than the biggest needle you have ever imagined poking into your gums. This book is meant to open your eyes ... or maybe more literally, to open your mouth. If you sense at any moment during your dental visit that something is not right, speak up and become part of the team. If your dentist keeps a schedule that presses you to "open up and shut up," be a little cautious (more to follow on those fast-paced dental offices and dentists who run behind schedule).

In the meantime, never be afraid to ask for second opinions. Your dentist is in all likelihood not evil, but may simply need more exposure to reality. He or she may, sadly, be in it for the money. You are not bound to one dentist, however, and if you are among the one in ten patients who have suffered pain or discomfort in the dental chair—get out of that chair. Find a dentist who listens, and whose passion is providing you with the best care possible. Again, only a very small number of dentists are out there causing more damage than good. If you are comfortable with your den-

This book is meant to open your eyes ... or maybe more literally, to open your mouth.

tist, you have probably made the right choice. Stick with them and create an ever stronger dentist-patient bond.

Obviously, I am just one dentist (with one team of qualified assistants), helping people in one specific location—I cannot fill all the cavities out there. But I can certainly use this book to guide you, the reader, and show what every visit to the dentist should look like. By covering the basics of dental care, the more complex choices, and the questions your dentist should be asking you— and vice versa—we will paint a picture featuring not just a pretty smile, but also a fundamentally healthy and empowering one. Let's also hope this book serves as a wakeup call for a few of the "bad" dentists out there to "open wide," and improve both their skills and their practice.

CHAPTER 2

Dental Care 101

YOU PROBABLY DON'T remember the pain you experienced when that very first tooth popped into your mouth at about six months of age, but you may have heard some stories about it. Maybe you grew up in the days before Baby Anbesol or baby aspirin, when parents and grandparents rubbed whiskey on your gums to numb the pain or calm you down.

Fast forward about six years, and you probably do remember losing your first tooth. As soon as that thing started to wiggle, you got excited. You would work on that tooth all day, always pushing it a little bit more with your fingers and tongue. One day you tasted blood, and you looked in the mirror and your loose tooth looked like it was dangling there by just a thread. Maybe your parents helped you with that final tug, tying one end of string around your tooth and the other end to a doorknob—and when they slammed the door shut, *voila*! You had survived a rite of passage. Then, of course, the Tooth Fairy visited you—leaving a coin or a dollar or some other small "prize" under your pillow while you slept.

The loss of childhood teeth holds joy and wonder—but of course, we spend the rest of our lives trying to retain all of our adult teeth.

Teeth have always held special powers. Today still, for better or for worse, we judge others on the condition of their teeth. Today, as technology advances and knowledge spreads, oral health in the United States continues to improve. People understand the importance of preventive care, and most know that a visit to the dentist at least every six months can help prevent more serious and costly dental visits down the road.

But a few sad facts persist: some people remain fearful, misinformed, or even ignorant when it comes to dental care. Some people wait years between dental visits, and even patients who know what is good for them report being lazy, or "forgetting" to follow basic, necessary oral hygiene routines. Most people know that oral hygiene involves taking care of their entire mouth—the gums, the teeth, the tongue, the cheeks, and so on. They know that oral hygiene begins with plaque removal, and that brushing and flossing their teeth more than once a day is crucial. But again—bad habits and misinformation persist. Even my best patients say to me some of the scariest things any dentist could hear:

- They think a yearly dental exam is enough.
- They make an appointment only when something hurts.
- When they are in pain or suspect oral infection, they take antibiotics they have lying around in their medicine cabinet.
- They are still using a medium or a hard toothbrush.

Fortunately, that last one, "I'm using a medium or hard brush because I really want to scrub my teeth clean," is the easiest one to remedy—before the patient even gets up from my chair. I end every visit by handing my patient a new soft toothbrush.

Clearly, the toothbrush has evolved, and consumers believe they have many options. "It's not true!" I tell my patients. "You *do not* have options when it comes to purchasing a toothbrush."

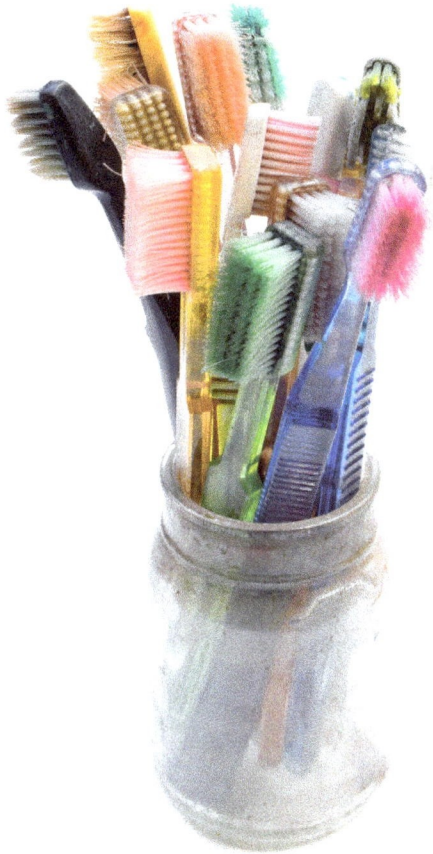

> The first thing I tell all my patients is this: Always buy a soft toothbrush.

The first thing I tell all my patients is this: Always buy a soft toothbrush. Contrary to logic, harder bristles do not do a better job of cleaning your teeth; in fact, they may cause a lot of damage. Medium- and hard-bristled brushes can damage your teeth and gums—sometimes irrevocably. The cleanliness of your teeth doesn't depend on *how hard* you brush them, but on *how well* you brush them. The only reason anyone should ever buy a medium- or hard-bristle toothbrush is to clean their dogs' teeth or to scrub the bathroom tile.

When choosing between a manual and an electric toothbrush, the electric toothbrush generally wins, and electric toothbrushes with round heads are better than those with rectangular heads because the circular shape forces you to brush one tooth at a time. Whether you prefer a manual or electric toothbrush, of course, is your choice—just always make sure it is soft.

If your gums are bleeding or sensitive at all, chances are something is wrong; possibly you are brushing your teeth incorrectly. If you are moving that brush back and forth or up and down like Ralph Macchio in the classic eighties film *The Karate Kid*—wax on, wax off—you are brushing wrong. If you aren't brushing your tongue morning and night—you guessed it—you aren't taking care of your mouth the way you need to. Brushing your teeth the wrong way (or with the wrong toothbrush) can lead to abrasions, plaque accumulation, gum recession, cavities, and so on. You know that famous saying, "He's grown long in the tooth"? Well, in dental circles, "long in the tooth" isn't just a euphemism for growing old; patients with too much tooth exposed, at any age, have been doing something wrong.

Brushing is only half of the equation. You must also floss properly.

Brushing your teeth the right way is simple and critical. The "Bass technique" of brushing, named after the dentist who invented it, is the best way to keep your pearly whites healthy and your gums in the best possible condition. If you've never heard of the Bass method before, the Internet has all the videos you need. Or better yet, ask your dentist to demonstrate. The Bass technique involves holding your brush at a forty-five-degree angle toward your gums, and moving it over your teeth in a tiny circular motion, applying light to moderate pressure. Working systematically, you should brush the outer surface of your teeth first, followed by the inner surface, and then the chewing surface.

The Bass technique is the most effective way to remove food particles and plaque from your mouth. Even patients with advanced gum disease are advised to use this method because it is safe, gentle, and effective. But using the Bass technique with a medium or hard toothbrush will do more harm than good.

Of course, brushing is only half of the equation. You must also floss properly. If you are unsure of what floss to buy and how to use it, talk to your dental hygienist or dentist—they should be happy to educate you. Again, brushing or flossing the incorrect way may cause irreversible damage.

Let me repeat: Buy a soft toothbrush and floss, get shown how to use them, then brush and floss, brush and floss, see your dentist, brush and floss.

Okay, at this point you may be thinking, "Wow, this dentist is obsessive about oral hygiene and soft toothbrushes!" You're right—I am. We are not sharks: we only get one set of adult teeth, so we must care for them with diligence. Think about the things most people obsess over. We put a lot of time into buying the car that best fits our needs, we purchase top-of-the-line appliances to improve our lives, and we research the exact right cell phone—and when we need to upgrade it all, we research again. We ask experts for advice on which running shoes best fit our feet, and we spend countless thousands of dollars on vitamins and gym memberships. We even buy anti-plaque treats for our cats and dogs. But when it comes to purchasing the most important piece of equipment we put in our mouths day in and day out, we choose willy-nilly.

One of my patients was resistant to switching to the soft toothbrush. He believed the hard bristles were doing a better job of cleaning his teeth. This patient was also not compliant with his regular check-ups, so by the time he finally made it in to see me, we discovered that he had been brushing so hard for so long with a hard toothbrush that he needed five root canals and five crowns. This client spent well over $9,000 for dental treatment that could very easily have been avoided.

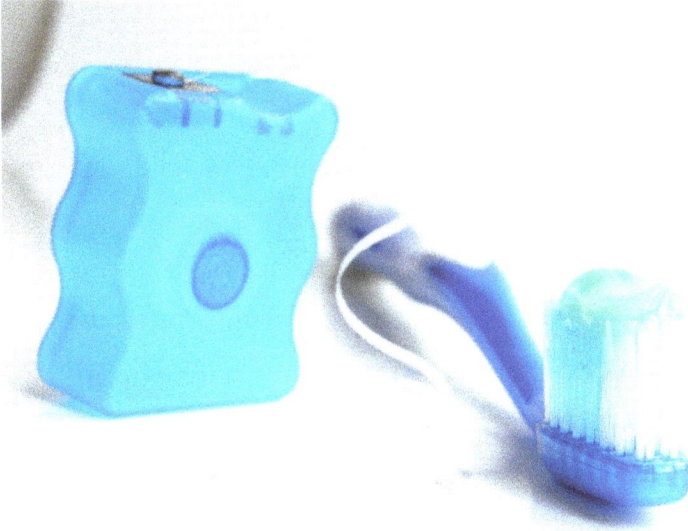

Like the toothbrush, toothpaste and dental floss have evolved too. Take a trip to your local drug store and stare down the dental aisle. Exciting, isn't it? Or is it overwhelming? There are flavored toothpastes, sparkling toothpastes, and ones that promise to remove tough stains like coffee and tobacco. There are flavored flosses, waxed and unwaxed flosses, nylon and monofilament flosses, dental floss picks, and more! You would think consumers were demanding just as much of the toothpaste and dental floss manufacturers as they demand of cell phone manufacturers. Whatever happened to the simple white goo you squeezed onto your soft brush and the string you pulled through your teeth after brushing?

Don't let that dental aisle intimidate you. Ask your dentist or hygienist which products they recommend (I happen to like

Colgate products). Also, most dentists will tell you that the best floss for you is the one you will use regularly. It's that simple. Follow a regular routine at home—it's an investment that will pay off. Your dentist knows if you aren't brushing and flossing regularly. Floss removes plaque (the thick, filmy coating that accumulates on your teeth), just as brushing does, but it also helps remove a type of bacteria brushing cannot remove—the kind that causes periodontal disease. Flossing prevents halitosis (bad breath) and gingival (gum) inflammation. Flossing takes no more than three minutes of your time, and it is a crucial part of your oral hygiene routine. Do you want bad breath and gum disease? If your answer is "no," then floss every day!

Daily brushing and flossing should help remove all plaque from your mouth. Plaque that remains in your mouth hardens and becomes *calculus*, which—trust me—is a lot worse than that difficult branch of mathematics so many teenagers dread in high school. When calculus is allowed to form and remain on your teeth for an extended period of time, bad breath, gum inflammation, and bone loss can occur. "Bone loss? I'm too young for that!" you say. Okay, but isn't bad breath scary enough? Don't you remember that calculus teacher, that favorite aunt, that friend's handsome father—who had bad breath? Don't be the person everyone takes one step back from. And don't take a chance on growing "long in the tooth" too soon, and destroying your fabulous smile.

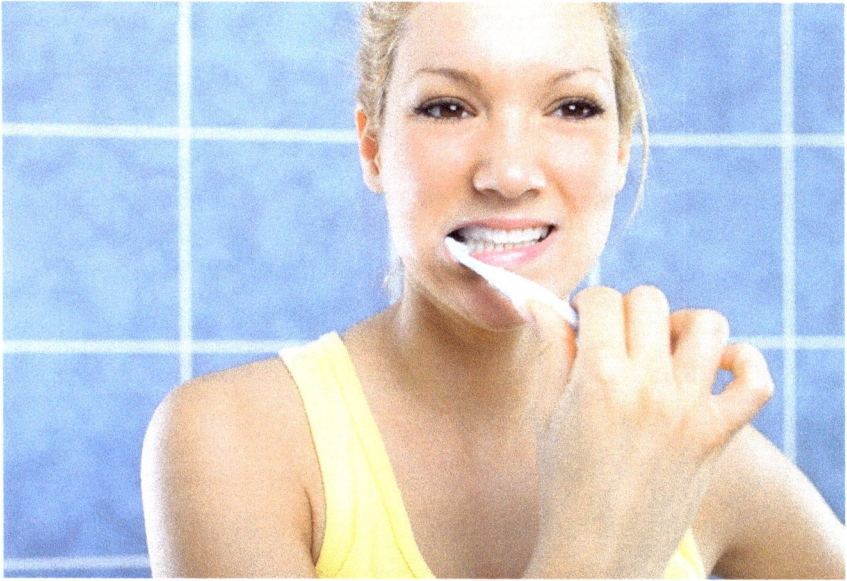

Most products in that dental aisle are your friend—the soft toothbrush, the antimicrobial mouth rinse, the floss that gets in there and glides best for you. Your dentist is your friend too, and you should always feel free to ask questions. Need to brush up on that Bass technique? Want to lean in and ask, "Do I have bad breath?" Did some Hollywood star's "secret to a winning smile" pop up in your social media feed? Do you want to know what you can do throughout the day, every day, to maintain a healthy, attractive mouth?

A good dentist never makes you feel rushed in the chair. A good dentist loves reviewing the basics of what you can and should do at home, between visits. In addition to brushing and flossing after every meal when you can, here are some quick tips for keeping most mouths fresh and happy throughout the day:

- *Chew gum after meals* (unless your dentist advises against it). This is a good thing to do as long as the gum is sugarless. Chewing gum stimulates your salivary flow, which acts as a buffer between the outer layer of your teeth and the harmful acids in much of your food.
- *Drink water after meals.* Drinking water after you eat helps wash food particles out of your mouth.
- *Avoid sticky foods and food or drinks that are high in sugar content.* Even though most dentists cringe at the thought of anybody drinking soda, we know everyone breaks down and has one from time to time. Keep in mind that most regular soda contains a ridiculously unhealthy amount of sugar, and that even diet sodas contain acidic substances that are bad for oral health. Speaking as a dentist, the best advice I can give patients who insist on drinking any kind of soda—one of the worst enemies of oral health—is this: finish it within ten minutes. In other words, don't sip your soda slowly over the course of an hour. Your saliva needs approximately twenty minutes to build the protective buffer mentioned above. If you prolong your soda intake, your mouth has to try to rebuild that buffer after every sip, giving

bacteria more time to settle in and stake its claim on your teeth. You think that television commercial with the green cartoon mucous guys is disgusting? Oral bacteria look just the same. I may sound like a broken record, but I really need to stress to all readers that I DO NOT recommend drinking soda.

- *Stay hydrated.* Think about the time you had one glass of wine too many and woke up with a pounding head. Remember the adjectives you used to describe your mouth. Remember how it felt like something "died in there?" Well, it had—your mouth was overloaded with bacteria. Drinking plenty of water is recommended by health practitioners of all kinds, and your dentist will tell you too: a hydrated mouth is a healthier mouth. If you don't have access to a toothbrush or a stick of gum, drink some water and take an extra gulp or two to rinse with. Even if you have to swallow that water, you have cleared some of the food particles from your teeth, and have thus reduced the amount of bacteria hanging around in your mouth causing nothing but odor and trouble.

Rather than lecture my patients, I try to keep them informed. After all, this is a long-term partnership, and unlike some dentists out there who charge for unnecessary treatments and procedures, I would rather see a hundred patients for their regular, affordable check-ups than see a few with serious, expensive issues. So much of what we do on a daily basis, and over the course of our lives, affects our health—and depends on our health. Our oral health affects us in the social, psychological, and professional realms, and the reason I practice dentistry is truly to give everyone an equal foot in the door—to enable more people to open doors with their smiles. When new patients come to me with a mouthful of cavities and exclaim, "But I never eat candy!" I don't eye them suspiciously. I'm a dentist, not the CIA. I say, "Hey, don't forget that other food sources turn to sugar during chemical breakdown," or, "Hey, many of the things we enjoy as adults—coffee, tea, wine, and soda—stain our teeth." Sometimes, it comes down to a very simple solution: I re-educate them on how to brush their teeth properly—with a soft toothbrush of course!

We are only human, we only live once, and I believe proper oral hygiene can help ensure more happiness. We are a fortunate nation in that our dental technology is some of the most advanced in the world. If we can combine what we know about the science of oral care with daily diligence and commitment to preventing all that gross, no-good bacteria from throwing a round-the-clock party in our mouths, we can all rest easier and wake up to much healthier smiles.

CHAPTER 3

You Have a Toothache.
What Should Your Dentist Do About It?

IF EVERY ONE of my patients saw me twice a year, the number of panicked, "Oh my God, something's wrong! Can I come in today?" phone calls my office receives would drop significantly. Pain and pain tolerance, of course, varies from person to person, but my rule is this: Don't wait until the pain is so bad you can't make it through another day. If you have any oral pain at all—any throbbing, tingling, or surges—treat it like you would treat chest pain. Get to a dentist as fast as you would go a doctor. Review your medical history with your dentist, and then get an x-ray and the proper prescription or treatment.

Sensitivity or pain in your mouth is a sign that something is wrong. You may have a small cavity that will cost less than $100 to treat, or you may need more expensive surgery that is outside your dentist's area of expertise and requires a referral. Either way, if you ignore your symptoms and hope for the best, things will get worse 100 percent of the time.

> Sensitivity or pain in your mouth is a sign that something is wrong. You may have a small cavity that will cost less than $100 to treat, or you may need more expensive surgery that is outside your dentist's area of expertise and requires a referral.

Compare your mouth to your car. You want it to be clean and comfortable and running at maximum efficiency at all times. When your engine needs oil, you take it to the shop, and they give you the $50 package deal and send you on your way. If you skip that simple oil maintenance for too long, your engine explodes, and then what are we talking about? Big dollars. We are talking about your car spending more time in the shop—inconveniencing you for a much longer period of time.

This is exactly how it works with oral hygiene and care: Just two visits to your dentist per year can potentially save you multiple visits per year—putting up with tooth pain for even one month too long often means you'll end up needing a root canal instead of possibly just a filling or a crown.

Most people are scared of needles; drills even more so. Your dentist puts his face in your face, and his gloved fingers pry your lips open and pull them this way and that. And what's with that little vacuum cleaner that—no matter where it is—gags you, grabs your tongue, and still lets drool roll off your chin? Patients aren't patient at all when it comes to the tools and gadgets and sounds and odors they must endure in the dentist's chair—but fear and loathing aside, not going to the dentist is just not an option.

Of course, the horror stories don't help. Everyone has heard about a dentist pulling a tooth with his knee on someone's chest (for the record, I have yet to meet a dentist who has ever done that). The power of social media, the Internet, and the human tendency to exaggerate make stories like this one easy to tell and retell. Some may be urban legends, and others may be true, but I urge you to find the right dentist and go regularly. Regular visits are necessary to ensure a healthy relationship with your dentist and to keep potential problems to a minimum.

How do you know if you have the wrong dentist … or a bad dentist? Since I happen to *be* a dentist, why would I write a book that calls other dentists out? Aren't I afraid that once this book hits the shelves, I'll be chased down the street by an angry army of my peers wielding huge hypodermics and rotten old pliers? First, the number of dentists in this category is small. Second, these practitioners may not know they are doing anything wrong. Finally, the purpose of this book is not to attack my peers maliciously. It is to raise awareness and to help elevate their level of care, which will in turn help both patients and practices to thrive.

> How do you know if you have the wrong dentist ... or a bad dentist?

So I'm just sharing with you what a high standard of care should look like. This begins with proper sterilization, practicing universal precautions, proper infection control, eliminating cross contamination, and following state laws regarding patient treatment. But these standards and practices must be understood by the patient in order for the relationship to be healthy for everyone. Understanding the dynamics of a dental office will provide you with better insight into the ultimate goal (this will be discussed as simply as possible in a later chapter).

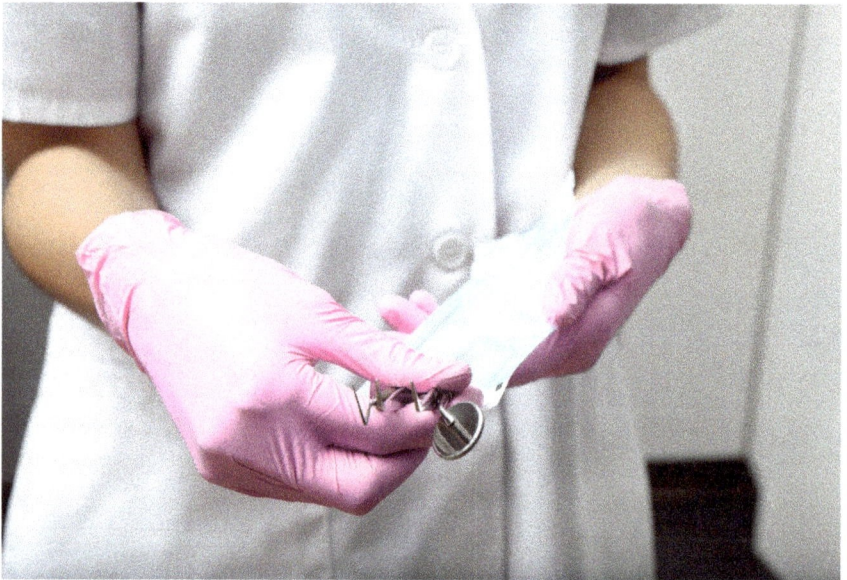

Going back to dental school would be a great place for all of us to start, because that's where we learned how to do everything the correct way. When we cut corners or don't follow instructions, proper care can be compromised.

But what's right and what's wrong? It is always wrong, for example, to skimp on sanitization. Picture your dentist putting that cute little mirror into your mouth—and imagine that just thirty minutes ago it was in some-one else's mouth, swabbed only with rubbing alcohol in between uses. Even if there's no blood or gum tissue on that mirror, there may still be plenty of bacteria. Rubbing alcohol can't remove bacterial spores from dental equip-ment—that is what your dentist's autoclave is for. An autoclave is a machine that sterilizes medical, dental, and laboratory equipment of all kinds using a high-pressure, highly-heated steam. Having a mirror in your mouth that has not been sterilized after every use is like going to a friend's house for dinner and finding out they are serving your dinner on a plate their dog has "cleaned" with his tongue.

> A dentist who does not sterilize equipment between each and every patient visit is either cutting financial corners or being lazy and saving himself time ... he or she is also endangering lives.

A dentist who does not sterilize equipment between each and every patient visit is either cutting financial corners or being lazy and saving himself time (the autoclave does wear down drills over time and requires at least thirty minutes to do its job), but he or she is also endangering lives. The mirror example may gross you out, but switch out that dental mirror with a dental drill that has not been properly sanitized, and now we are talking about the possible transfer of blood and blood-borne diseases and viruses such as hepatitis, tuberculosis, and HIV.

Indeed, in the early nineties, the well-known investigation of Dr. David Acer, a dentist who had infected six of his patients with the HIV virus, was cut short when he died of AIDS. Experts, staff, and people who knew him are still unable to understand how he infected his patients, and some wonder whether he may have done it on purpose. Either way, a quote from a June 6, 1993, *New York Times* article (one of the many *Times* articles written about the case) supports my point—many dentists cut corners when it comes to sanitization: "Investigators said Dr. Acer did not always sterilize his equipment, but that he was no more sloppy than other dentists in the area."

"Sloppy?" How about *deadly*?

Fortunately—and I use that word reluctantly—not all sloppy or bad dentistry produces such horrific results. The majority of patient neglect cases I have seen over the years involve work done on the wrong tooth, or the wrong kind of work done on the right tooth—but either way, wrong work ultimately means more pain and more expense for the patient. The sad thing is, most mistakes could have been and should have been prevented, but because the dentist was rushed or tired or lazy or distracted, the mistake was made.

In carpentry, the rule is "measure twice, cut once." A carpenter who keeps cutting a home's wallboards even a half inch too short will eventually be fired. Or worse, he'll finish the job and deliver an unsafe and unsound house. When you go to your dentist with a toothache, there is a specific protocol that dentist should follow. We are not comparing dentistry to carpentry here;

just emphasizing the common need to be precise. Without the proper medical history and diagnostic tools, and without a precise treatment plan, a lot can go wrong.

I don't know how many people I have treated have told me about a former dentist who took them in, sat them in the chair, asked, "Where's the pain?" and then went to work drilling or extracting a tooth. Crazy, right? Well let's flip the script here. A patient calls screaming bloody murder, in so much pain that she needs to be seen immediately. The scheduling coordinator gets her in right away. Meanwhile the dentist already has a patient in the chair, and he's having trouble getting fully anesthetized. In addition, two of his hygienists are waiting for an examination and his next scheduled patient has arrived. Although the dentist most likely doesn't have enough time to see the emergency patient, the appointment is scheduled anyway. That emergency patient has been a patient of record for twenty years, and she is very loyal. This patient is truly in need of care and rightfully should be seen.

Now the stress level is elevating throughout the office. The emergency patient arrives and is waiting patiently, but tears are welling up because she is in extreme pain. Both waiting patients are quickly seated. Within five minutes the dentist looks at the emergency patient, sees that the tooth needs to be removed, and has his assistants prepare for an extraction. He goes into the other treatment room and tends to his regularly scheduled patient while the dental assistant gets consent for the extraction.

Within the next ten minutes the dentist returns to the emergency patient, anesthetizes her, and quickly removes the tooth.

Tears of joy now come from the patient. When things slow down a little, the dentist asks to have the x-ray sent to the insurance company for payment. The assistant looks at him with a blank stare. No x-ray was taken! Although the lack of an x-ray did not have a major negative effect on overall treatment, things like this can and do happen. A good lesson would be if you are in this situation and know that an x-ray is necessary, don't be afraid to ask. Also, if you understand the dynamics of a dental office, you will look at your appointments differently.

I often hear about cases in which a dentist puts a filling in, say, tooth #12, only to discover a week later, after continued and worsening pain—and finally, an x-ray—that tooth #13 was actually the tooth with the cavity. Talk about adding insult to injury! How would you feel if one of your perfectly healthy teeth were drilled and filled, or even extracted, for no good reason at all?

People should get upset reading this book, but more important, they should be informed about how they can help prevent these kinds of problems. My goal is not to lay a pretty veneer over the truth about bad dentistry. Bad dentistry is sometimes as obvious as a bad veneer, but much more often, sadly, it is not obvious at all. Short of a dentist being honest enough to say, "Sorry, I have to tell you I made a mistake in your mouth last week," you may never be aware of the dental work you've had done that you did not need … unless or until it goes horribly wrong! I have much more respect—and so should you—for the dentist who admits his or her mistakes.

Unless a funny feeling afterward motivates you to go in for a second opinion, and x-rays show that the five fillings your new dentist just "urgently" gave your young son were completely unnecessary, you might never doubt that the next $500 worth of procedures he insists on are necessary. Unless you have a cousin who is completing her dental school internship hours, and who sees you and says, "A chipped front tooth? That could have been taken care of with white filling for under $300," you won't know that the greedy dentist who said your only option was $5,000 worth of veneers on all six front teeth was more concerned with his pool payments than your oral health.

The above stories are true, and so are other stories of dentists who failed to review their patients' medical histories and prescribed dangerous or lethal medications (or failed to prescribe medication when it was needed). A dentist who prescribes certain antibiotics to a patient who is allergic to those antibiotics is a careless and dangerous dentist. A dentist who does not pre-medicate (give medication prior to performing a dental procedure) a patient with an organ transplant puts that patient's life at risk. Again, I stress the importance of knowing your medical conditions and sharing them fully with your dentist. He can't alter your treatment if he doesn't have the facts.

You are asked a few basic questions every time you go to your regular medical doctor. You are weighed, your blood pressure is taken, and so on. When you go to your dentist, be sure you are being asked if anything in your medical history has changed since your last visit. If no one asks, just volunteer the information. Tell

Communication between you and your dentist should be continually updated, and you should never feel rushed.

them of any changes, regardless of what those changes may be. Tell them you are happy to report that your complete physical and blood results were unremarkable. Communication between you and your dentist should be continually updated, and you should never feel rushed.

If you need to give your dentist that panic call ("It hurts!"), you hope he will find time to see you as soon as possible. When I receive such calls, I run a quick triage: On a scale of one to ten, ten being the most painful, how much does it hurt? Is there any swelling? Are you having difficulty swallowing or breathing? Often, I will offer to take a quick look at no charge—because it can be dangerous for a patient to think, *I'll only go in when it hurts.* The more dangerous the emergency is to my patient or the more it hurts, the faster I get them in. Increased pain and sensitivity tell me that the protective enamel has been compromised by bacteria, and that bacteria could travel to the nerve, which may lead to infection, an abscess, or to an otherwise dangerous situation.

By no means am I saying that your "quick" visits should be free of charge. Dentists complete extensive training to be able to quickly diagnose problems and pathology. Of course they should be fairly compensated for their treatment and their time.

Another important point about x-rays: Do not fear the x-ray; fear the dentist who insists they aren't necessary. Each of the above stories of patients whose teeth were wrongly filled or removed is the result of a dentist who either did not take new x-rays or did not review existing ones before tooling up. X-rays allow the dentist to detect problems that cannot be seen with the clinical eye. Small cavities, cracks, or chips between the teeth, as well as bone pathologies and oral cancers, can be seen only via x-ray. Any "dangers" you might fear regarding x-rays are always outweighed by the benefits. Technology has improved, and the radiation received from a complete set of dental x-rays is equivalent to spending just a couple of hours in the sun or taking an airline flight.

> If you find your dentist's waiting room too cold or too hot, too gloomy or too bright— ask yourself, "Is there something wrong here?" If the staff look and act miserable, or your dentist comes in with bad breath and bad teeth and an itch he just can't seem to scratch, trust your gut instincts.

Sure, the lowest of the low practitioners out there will always find *something* wrong with your teeth, as in the case with the young boy who "suddenly" had five cavities—but who in reality, had none. If you find your dentist's waiting room too cold or too hot, too gloomy or too bright—ask yourself, "Is there something wrong here?" If the staff look and act miserable, or your dentist comes in with bad breath and bad teeth and an itch he just can't seem to scratch, trust your gut instincts. When it comes to finding a dentist you can trust, don't trust everything you read on the Internet—go to the source. Find a few patients you can survey. Look at their teeth, and ask them if they are happy or unhappy, and why.

Consider whether your dentist's schedule will work with yours—if you know your best appointment time will usually be 7:00 in the evening, perhaps it would be wise to find a dentist who doesn't start at 7:00 a.m.—because even the best dentist in the world may get careless at the last appointment of a twelve-hour day.

I would like to believe there are thousands of dentists nationwide just like me who care about people more than they care about money. When you care about people, the money will come—that happy patient with the healthy mouth is going to recommend you to her aunt, her uncle, her mother, and her friends and colleagues. In all cases, from regular checkups to urgent situations, my patients know my office is open for free tours, and not just to potential patients. When I was a kid, that's what my dentist offered, and taking that tour influenced the course of my life. I'm not saying a friendly visit to the dentist will turn everyone into lifelong dental fanatics, but if a visit to my office or a visit to the pages of this book helps to educate people about dentistry, it's worth it.

I'm not suggesting you keep digging until you find one little thing wrong at your dentist's office and go running for the hills. I urge readers simply to pay good attention during their next dental visit. If you are comfortable and happy, stay with your dentist and don't look for something to go wrong. Your gut tells you most of what you need to know. Trust it, and trust your dentist.

CHAPTER 4

Are You Getting All the Options You Deserve? Choices and Treatment Plans

WE DENTISTS ARE aware of our reputation—we are, to many, the scary tool-wielding torturers of your nightmares! We know people delay or avoid their recommended twice-yearly check ups, thinking that it will save them money—when in reality, *not* coming in is what will cost them. Cost? Oh yes, we know people would much rather spend their $2,000 Christmas bonus on a vacation in the tropics than on a root canal. We go to parties, and we know everyone has a dental horror story that gets passed around. We even know that we are never voted Most Popular among our medical peers.

My hope is that this book will convince people that none of the above circumstances have to be true. I hope that even if readers do not come to love their dentists, they will at least be able to assess whether their dentist is as ethical, as thorough, and as safe as they expect and need him or her to be. And I hope that this book will raise readers' awareness and expectations when it comes to dentistry, and that they will acquire a better understanding of My team is trained to treat each and every one of our patients

My hope is that this book will convince people that none of the above circumstances have to be true. I hope that even if readers do not come to love their dentists, they will at least be able to assess whether their dentist is as ethical, as thorough, and as safe as they expect and need him or her to be.

as if they were our own family members or close friends—what kind of dental experience would they want and expect? Every dentist and every dental team should ask themselves the same question, and should deliver the highest level of care to every patient. Every dentist—including your dentist—should be earning your trust at every visit.

So how do you know if your dentist is trustworthy? How do you know he or she is truly concerned about your overall health? How can you be sure you won't be given a "Band-Aid" treatment that will land you right back in the chair before the year ends?

We have already touched upon the crucial need for a full disclosure, review, and update of your medical history. We have stressed the importance of trusting your gut instincts about the environment in the waiting room and in the dental chair. We have implied, I hope, that there are no stupid questions when it comes to your oral health and hygiene—if you are unclear on the best way to brush, just ask for a demonstration.

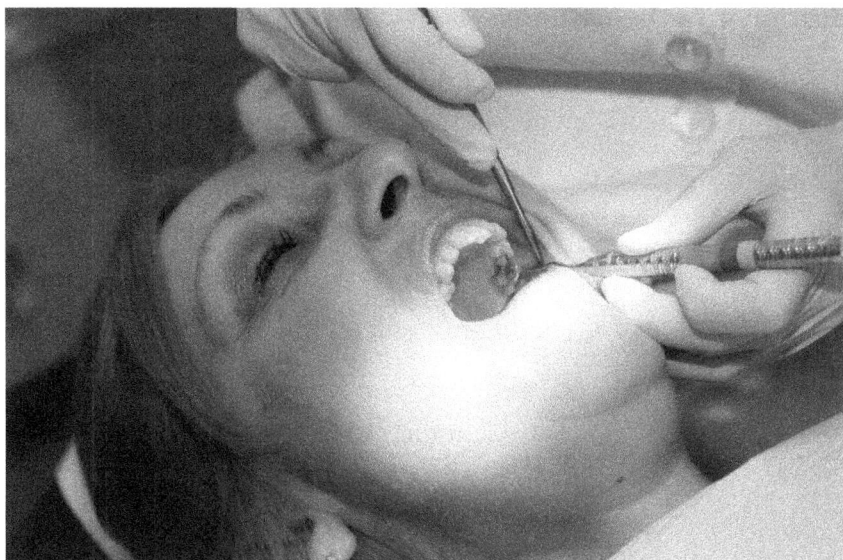

• • •

In this chapter, I want to delve deeper into what it means to have choices as a dental patient, and how to evaluate whether or not your dentist is presenting you with all the suitable treatment options when a problem presents itself. If you are practicing good home care and have a good diet, you will often find that when you come in for your routine checkup all you need is a routine cleaning, a "thumbs up," and you are good to go. If you are less fortunate or if your home care needs work, your dentist may discover a cavity, decay, gingivitis, halitosis, signs of periodontal disease, or any number of problems

> Every dentist— including *your* dentist—should be earning your trust at every visit.

that need immediate attention. You'll listen carefully, and hopefully you'll ask, "What are my options?"

Your dentist should present the best option first, the one that best meets the high standards of quality care—the option that he or she would use on his or her own mother or child. If money were no issue, what work would you have done? Of course, money *is* an issue, and one of the messages of this book is to take care that you are not misled into expensive and unnecessary treatment. There are bad apples in every field, as we all know, and even if just one percent of dentists are shady, it can make it a real challenge for the patient to know who to trust with their hard-earned money (not to mention their mouth).

• • •

The best dentists, as I've said, present you first with the treatment plan they would want for themselves. For example, those four large cavities you have on your back teeth should be filled with ceramic—the most durable and aesthetically pleasing of your three options for fillings in the back teeth. Do you *need* ceramic on your back teeth if you can't afford it? Will anyone notice if you have composite that far back in your mouth? These are all questions you should feel free to ask. Your dentist should never ignore or invalidate your concerns, whether they are basic oral health questions, aesthetic issues, or financial realities. If a service or procedure that is offered is one that you cannot possibly afford, a good dental office will walk you through possible financing options, including a third-party lender. A good dentist—your dentist—does not want to break your bank. But above all, a good dentist does not want to see you go another week without the care you need.

Your needs—your overall health needs, your oral health needs, and your bigger "life" needs—should be on your mind every single time you visit your dentist. If composite fillings prove to be the right solution for those four large cavities, a good dentist won't deny it. If a porcelain/metal crown will do for one tooth, but you need all-porcelain crowns on two others, your dentist should offer that information freely. That said, if you come in wanting your teeth whitened

> Your dentist should never ignore or invalidate your concerns, whether they are basic oral health questions, aesthetic issues, or financial realities. If a service or procedure that is offered is one that you cannot possibly afford, a good dental office will walk you through possible financing options, including a third-party lender.

and straightened, but your dentist finds decay and you need a root canal, beware if he says he will attend to your cash-specific *wants* before your health-specific *needs*. Again, a good dentist will never prioritize the flash of your smile over the holistic picture of your health.

> Again, a good dentist will never prioritize the flash of your smile over the holistic picture of your health.

Oral decay can lead to various health problems. Bacteria in the mouth can cause heart and stomach problems, infection, and more. When your dentist finds a problem, it is his or her job to explain that problem and its consequences: You have a hole in your tooth; disease will get in. You may then ask what your options are—and in many cases, you'll learn there is a range of options. If your dentist treats every single problem with the cheapest option, beware. That cheapest treatment may break down in five months, and the money you believe you are saving will ultimately come due. Alternately, if your dentist tells you, "It's the most expensive way or the highway, too bad you just lost your job and your dog had a $5,000 vet bill," consider that a warning sign too.

None of this is to say that the "middle road" is always the best road to take when considering your oral health needs. Different patients have different medical histories and different current life circumstances. A good dentist respects the entire picture, but never sacrifices what he or she upholds as a best practice. Dentists need dental treatment too, and the best of us "do unto others as we would have done to ourselves."

This is another opportunity for you as a patient to help create a healthy solution. Talk with your dentist and let him know what your expectations are, and the solution usually comes much more easily for both of you. As the song goes, you can't always get what you want. For example: a patient may "want" just a filling on a tooth that ends up requiring a root canal and crown. He won't get the filling, and the dentist will explain why.

The best dentists value getting to know their patients over the long term, and out of that comes an ability to read oddities in the record when they appear. If we see that one of our regular middle-aged patients experiencing a spike in the number of cavities, we will take the time to sit down and review what may have changed recently in his or her diet and lifestyle.

Remember, despite our reputation as drill-happy brutes, most dentists delight in being able to offer commonsense, easy-to-implement tips and solutions to our patients. If at any moment you feel unhappy or unsure about either the simple advice or the complicated treatment plan your dentist is offering, feel free to speak up.

If your dentist suggests changing your treatment plan mid-stream, or draws out the plan for a surprising length of time—ask why. Get answers! A good dentist knows all he or she needs to know before going in to perform any procedure. That dentist has reviewed your medical history, has taken new x-rays, and has discussed the problem with you, as well as the consequences of inaction and your treatment options. And you have agreed with him or her on a best course of action—prior to taking that action. Any dentist who "suddenly discovers" there is a lot more to be done may not have been extremely thorough with the exam and diagnosis. This does happen. What's important is that the correct treatment is ultimately provided. Of course, in dentistry

> Do not forget that one of the most important parts of your treatment plan includes what you must do to take care of yourself after you leave your dentist's office. You should know precisely what level of post-treatment swelling or discomfort is to be expected.

not everything goes 100 percent as expected. A deep filling may turn into a root canal or a crown. But if something seems far afield from the original treatment plan, feel free to raise an eyebrow—and again, ask why.

Do not forget that one of the most important parts of your treatment plan includes what you must do to take care of yourself after you leave your dentist's office. You should know precisely what level of post-treatment swelling or discomfort is to be expected. All prescribed post-treatment medications should not only be double-checked against your most recent medical records, but should also be taken only as prescribed. Just as we stress to our patients the importance of keeping up with their brushing and flossing, we stress to anyone who comes to us with a problem the importance of following through on the work he or she has just undergone. Patients should look at prescriptions as another part of the team approach. If you know you have an allergy to penicillin and your dentist prescribes it, by all means speak up. Become an integral player and say you need something else, then ask them to note it in your chart. Rather than getting upset because the wrong medication was prescribed, take pride in the fact that you're participating in the solution.

* * *

Understanding treatment planning is also important for patients. When your car needs new tires, you don't change just one. If you need heart surgery, you probably won't go to the first surgeon you find under "Heart Surgeons," in the phone book, or on the internet, and you won't schedule just one chamber to be repaired. The same goes for your mouth. Dental professionals strive to provide the treatment that will last the longest and be the safest, while eliminating all pathology. If a patient needs three fillings, two crowns, and a cleaning, but says he only wants the cleaning and the fillings, some type of pathology still exists. This may lead to further pathology, poor function, and possibly future pain. The goal is to complete all treatment in a timely manner. So thinking that you can do half of the treatment today and postpone the rest until next year may not be wise. This is another team-building opportunity. Following through with each and every step of that plan is crucial—why invest in a Cadillac if you're only going to give it the cheapest gas and let it collect dust, rust, and crust? Even the least expensive treatment plan needs to be well begun and then seen fully through.

Chapter 5

Is Your Dentist's Office
Hazardous to Your Health?

I WISH STORIES like the following were not true, but unfortunately they are.

In Fall River, Massachusetts, a former dentist was sentenced to a year in jail for using paper clips instead of stainless steel posts in root canals. He eventually pleaded guilty to assault and battery, defrauding Medicaid of $130,000, illegally prescribing medications, and witness intimidation. Prosecutors said he had been suspended by Medicaid in 2002, but continued to file claims until June 2005, using the names of other dentists in his practice. His license to practice dentistry in Massachusetts was suspended in 2006, and he is no longer licensed to practice dentistry in any state.

Since early 2013, Oklahoma health officials have set out to test 7,000 patients of one local dentist after one of his patients, who had no known risk factors, tested positive for hepatitis C. This case led to a surprise investigation of the Tulsa dental office, which revealed the use of rusty tools and sanitation equipment that hadn't been tested in six years. In addition, former employees testified to being forced to re-use needles and to use bleach to treat wounds in patients' mouths. As this book goes to press, of the several thousand patients who have been tested (along with their spouses and partners), eighty-nine have tested positive for hepatitis C, five for hepatitis B, and four for HIV. The dentist, who had been in practice for close to four decades, was labeled a "menace to public health," and voluntarily gave up his license.

These may seem like extreme cases straight out of a Hollywood horror film, but sadly they are fact, not fiction. The best dentists never work below a certain set of MANDATORY health and safety standards, which are known as the Universal Precautions.

If your dentist walks into your room wearing gloves, you might think everything is okay … until he walks right past you to the sink and washes his hands with those gloves still on—the ones he wore while working on another patient. Pulling a tray of instruments out of the autoclave could be a good thing, but are those tools bagged? Does your dentist open the sealed bag of sterilized tools in front of you? If he is working on you and finds he is missing a tool, does he reach over and open a drawer and pull one out of that drawer—cross-contaminating everything he touches? What if you were told that

> The best dentists never work below a certain set of MANDATORY health and safety standards, which are known as the Universal Precautions.

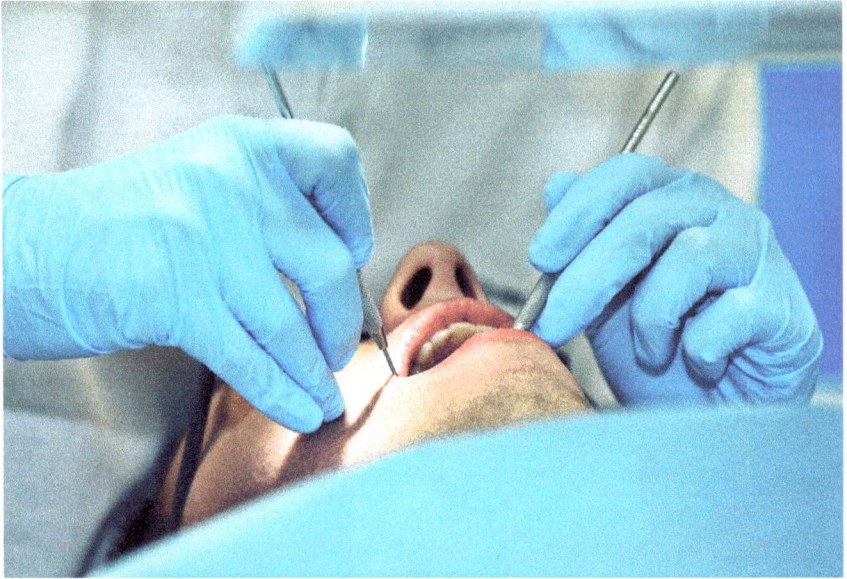

a real dentist—me, the guy writing this book—bought a retiring dentist's office only to discover that the guy didn't even have an autoclave … but that he did have a toaster oven? This is only funny if the guy wasn't *your* dentist.

Have you ever sat in an overcrowded waiting room, overhearing complaints about how late your dentist was running? Did it worry you a little? Did you wonder why your dentist wasn't respecting your time? Did you ask yourself how he and his team found the time to clean instruments between patients if appointments were so tightly packed? Did your gut tell you that wasting time reading magazines you would never subscribe to, and then being rushed into and out of the dental chair, was somehow robbing you of a chance to ask your dentist a few questions?

It's great that you are beginning to think on a different level, but we need to remember the team approach. First let's think about the doctor's office. Have you ever waited? I've actually considered packing lunch to go to a doctor's appointment. I always wondered why they booked me for 1:00 p.m. and took me in to the treatment room at 2:15, only to have me wait another fifteen minutes for the doctor to show up. We don't want you feeling like you need to bring pajamas to a dental appointment, but it sometimes happens that patients have to wait a few minutes—even up to forty-five minutes. Sometimes there is an emergency, a filling that goes worse than expected and turns into a root canal, or even a three-second break to take a drink of water; small delays like this can add up over the course of a day.

Things do not always go as planned in the dental office. How about when the office manager has to leave to pick up her son from school because he's sick? How about a medical doctor calling to discuss a patient who is scheduled in thirty minutes? That call may take an additional ten minutes out of the day. This is the perfect opportunity to discuss why you, the patient, should always be early, or at the very least on time. Because if the dentist has a day like that and three of his patients show up ten or fifteen minutes late, the office will be complete chaos.

But am I saying it's okay for the dentist to be late but it's not okay for the patient to be late? That's exactly what I am saying. Once this is understood, the relationship between the patient and the team becomes even stronger.

Getting back to office standards, no dentist I know, including myself, wants patients thinking they have to bring their own gloves and tools to the dental office. The idea is not to increase your fear of visiting your dentist twice yearly. Again, this book is in your hands now to raise awareness—yours as well as that of your family, friends, and colleagues. My goal is to emphasize that there is a right way and a wrong way of doing dentistry, and by reading some of the more shocking truths about the wrong way, hopefully you will be steered quickly toward dentists who will treat you with as much care and respect as they would their own family.

There are no regular dental office inspections to ensure that proper sterilization techniques are being used. OSHA, the Occupational Safety and Health Administration, usually won't send someone to inspect except in insurance audit cases, when a legal matter arises, or—as in the case of the bad dentist in Tulsa, Oklahoma—under unusual circumstances. In general, OSHA trusts that dentists have ethics, and most do. But when a dentist

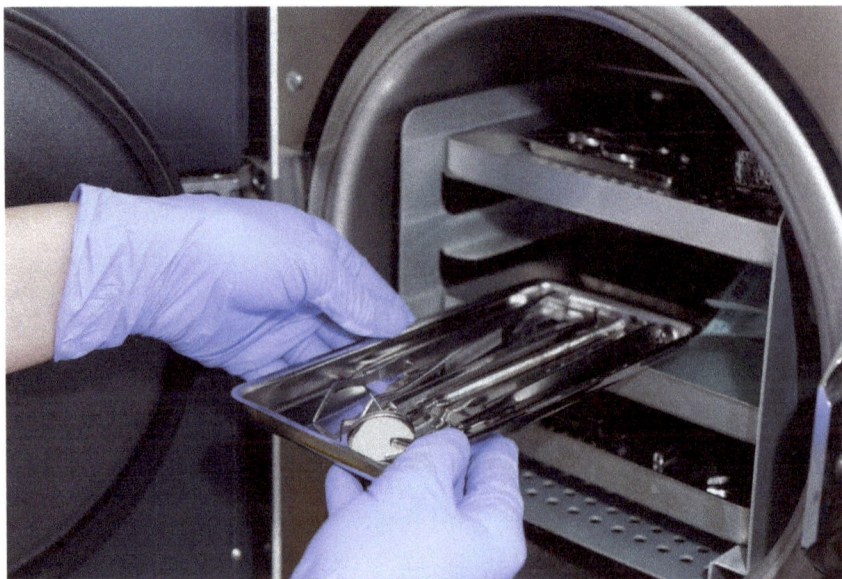

and his or her team slack on ethics, every patient who sits in that
chair faces a life or death situation.

Autoclaves, as I've said, are
the only machines that guarantee proper sterilization of dental
tools, because they use highly
pressurized steam.

The retiring dentist whose
office I bought should have
known that dry heat from a

> A good dentist
> checks his or her
> autoclave on a
> regular basis by
> using testing strips,
> which are sent out
> of office and given
> a "pass" or "fail."

toaster oven could never guarantee patient safety and health—
and certainly I prefer to think he didn't know, rather than that
he didn't care. Yes, autoclaves are expensive and require main-
tenance, but any dentist worth seeing knows there is no other
option. A good dentist checks his or her autoclave on a regular
basis by using testing strips, which are sent out of office and
given a "pass" or "fail." Good dentists and good dental teams
make sure the sterilization bags that hold the tools turn the color
they are supposed to turn, indicating that the contents of the
bags are sterile and safe for patients.

A good dentist also invests in enough tools—so that in the
rare event that there is a backlog of appointments (don't forget:
the good dental office tries its best to schedule well), there is never
the temptation to rush a set of instruments through the autoclave—or worse, to ignore the required sanitation procedures
between patients. A good dentist also knows that rusty tools,

A good dentist also invests in enough tools—so that in the rare event that there is a backlog of appointments (don't forget: the good dental office tries its best to schedule well), there is never the temptation to rush a set of instruments through the autoclave—or worse, to ignore the required sanitation procedures between patients.

like the ones used by the dentist in Tulsa, cannot be sterilized even with a properly functioning autoclave.

Regulations vary statewide (it is not required by law to bag instruments), but if your dentist is not opening a bag of sterilized instruments in front of you, feel free to ask if the instruments were properly sterilized. You don't need to drill your dentist, but if you inspect the cuspidor—that white bowl next to the chair you are asked to spit in during a cleaning—and it looks like a homicide scene, please do question your dentist's sanitation standards … as you are running out the door!

Know too that sterilization involves more than just the autoclave. From the moment you are seated to the moment you step out the door, you can potentially come into contact with the saliva, blood, and gum tissue of other patients. If you see any signs that your chair, the cuspidor, or the trays have not been sprayed down and wiped clean before you take your place, speak up. If you feel at all intimidated to ask questions, think of how bacteria breed and transfer from hand to hand and from hand to mouth—that should help you prioritize your concerns.

Your dentist's job is to protect everyone in his or her circle. This involves hiring reputable dental assistants with radiology licenses and good credentials—not just any Craigslist job seeker. The responsibility to protect everyone

> Your dentist and everyone on his or her team needs to treat every patient who walks in the door as if that patient were carrying a communicable disease.

in the dental circle extends beyond the office to include technicians at outside labs. Before the impression for a crown gets sent out, a good dental team sprays that impression with an antimicrobial spray.

Infection control is the name of the game, and if your dentist is reusing equipment or simply wiping drills down between patients, your life is at risk—and frankly, so are the lives of everyone in that office. Even the tiniest, most invisible particle from between the grooves of a small drill bit can spread disease or even kill.

Conversely, your dentist and everyone on his or her team needs to treat every patient who walks in the door as if that patient were carrying a communicable disease. This is not a judgment of character; this is meant to ensure maximum protection for potentially

> When you find the right dentist, you'll find comfort in that chair.

thousands of people. You may be the cleanest-cut, wealthiest, and fittest guy on your block, but you could still be carrying HIV, hepatitis, or some other blood-borne or airborne disease. The best dentists, as I said earlier, are trained from day one to practice Universal Precaution and infection control standards, and those practices should be automatic.

An ethical dental office's standards also cover the dissemination of critical post-operative instructions. If your dentist pulls a tooth and says nothing but, "We got it! See you later!" you should be worried. Even if you were in two weeks prior to have a tooth pulled, and the week before that to have a second tooth pulled, on that third visit—yes, on each and every visit—you should be given verbal and written post-op instructions. You should also be instructed to call your dentist should any oral pain, swelling, or black and blue discoloration occur. This is another area where the team approach will come into play. After having a procedure that you are unfamiliar with (like an extraction), ask what you should do or not do so you can avoid any potential problems.

When you find the right dentist, you'll find comfort in that chair. Don't shake your head or laugh; it is possible! Your dentist and dental team are not practicing dental care for their own health, but for yours. Dentists who are invested in their profession *do* care, and they appreciate clients who show up on time, slide into that chair with confidence, and pay attention. Open your eyes wide the next time you visit your dentist, and assess whether or not you feel absolutely sure of your surroundings. If you are unsure, speak up. If you like what you see, lean back, close your eyes, and open wide.

CHAPTER 6

Is Your Dentist Qualified to Run a Practice?

NOT EVERY KID knows, like I did at age twelve, that they want to grow up to be a dentist. Very early on, I had an interest in teeth—and a great dentist who enjoyed giving me tours of his office and educating me as much as he could educate a kid my age. In high school, in anticipation of attending dental school, I loaded up on biology and chemistry courses. I took three years of college courses and transferred to dental school. Now, several decades into my practice, I continue to attend seminars and training sessions in order to keep myself abreast of the latest trends and advances in the art and science of dentistry.

Right out of dental school, though, I worked with several dentists whose lack of ethics shocked me. It wasn't that I was naïve or idealistic, but I didn't expect the people I was working with to employ the sorts of careless and dangerous practices and procedures I witnessed on a regular basis.

• • •

Most dental school graduates start out in debt, and with little if any experience running the business end of a practice, so we spend several years working with other dentists until we are ready to open our own offices. I worked for six or eight dentists in my mid to late twenties. Not long into my employment with one dentist, I witnessed him doing something very disturbing, which became even more disturbing when I realized it was part of his daily routine. This dentist had a ten-ounce container of polishing paste, and he used the paste in that cup all day long—every day, with a roster of nearly a dozen patients. Despite the fact that individual packets of polishing paste were available, or that this dentist could have used smaller cups and portions throughout the day, he dipped in and out of that cup and in and out of various patients' mouths, seeming not to care at all about cross-contamination.

I was just as mortified when another dentist with whom I worked told me to "find something wrong ... anything" with one of his patients. A sixteen-year-old girl was in the chair, and when she asked me when she needed to return for more work, I responded, "You're good to go." This dentist, who until that point had impressed me as one of the good guys, said, "No, no, no! You have to find *something* wrong. She hasn't been here in over a year." I looked at the dentist and shrugged. *Nothing* was wrong with this young girl's oral health. Nevertheless, the dentist proceeded to give her a second lookover, after which he announced that she had five cavities. "Make the appointment and do the work on her," I was told.

Dental school had not prepared me for this kind of dilemma. I was twenty-six years old and still gaining experience. So there I stood, in my inexperienced shoes, at the mercy of my employer, saying, "If you can show me decay in the x-rays, I'll do the fillings; but if not, you do them." It was one of my first exposures to pure greed in the dental field, but unfortunately, it wasn't my last—not until I opened my own practice and was able to establish and maintain my own high standards regarding my work.

> The truth is that there is no policing body in dentistry. Nobody is looking over our shoulders ensuring that we are following ethical codes.

The truth is that there is no policing body in dentistry. Nobody is looking over our shoulders ensuring that we are following ethical codes. When you get out of dental school, you can do almost anything—you can decide to stay in general dentistry or go on for more schooling. After another three years after dental school, for example, you can specialize in endodontics; another six years, and you can become a dental surgeon. Taking any continuing education coursework once we are set up in our practice is solely up to each of us. Just as with any profession, there are stellar dentists, decent dentists, and despicable dentists—and again, that is why I am writing this book: to help you recognize the difference.

During those early years, when I witnessed some dentists ordering cheap supplies and using cheap labs, I came to understand how bad business practices could lead one down an ethically questionable path.

As soon as it was financially possible, I began to take continuing education courses in the field of dentistry. Since opening my own practice nearly two decades ago, I have invested tens of thousands of dollars in business management courses—and frankly, I don't see how some of my peers get by without learning these skills. When I think back to my earliest days, when I was bringing in $2,000 a day but paying $1,700 right back out in overhead, I'm glad I realized early on the value in studying dentistry as a business. During those early years, when I witnessed some dentists ordering cheap supplies and using cheap labs, I came to understand how bad business practices could lead one down an ethically questionable path. I decided that what cost me now would save and make me more money later. I knew that if I started with the best materials, the best labs, the best staff, and the best business practices, people would hear about it and choose me. My business grew quickly, and it continues to grow today.

Taking courses in practice management, however, is just one piece of the ongoing continuing education process. Dental science moves fast. If you are out of the loop for five or ten years, you will be behind. Keeping up with the dental news coming out of New York and California, where they seem at times to be light years ahead of the rest of the nation and the world, keeps me current with the latest and greatest in dentistry.

Science and coursework are of course just two pieces of the overall dentistry picture. Even if I have stayed on top of the science—learning about the latest and best new materials, and turning my office into a mean, lean money-wise machine—that still isn't enough. Dentistry is an art, and your dentist-as-artist should

> In fact, dentists really shouldn't be touting themselves as jacks-of-all-trades. ... As a patient, it is truly not in your best interest to beg your dentist, no matter how much you admire and respect him or her, to do work he or she is saying "No" to.

be deeply into the work he or she does. The best of us are proud to know our own art is on display more than any Picasso or Van Gogh ever will be. The best dentists find and use the best labs—labs that also consider their work to be artistic. Our patients are our walking billboards—their smiles say it all. There are no "non-cosmetic" dentists, because all dentistry involves beauty—we help make your mouth cleaner, healthier, and more attractive.

My duty and my passion are to care about my patients' oral health. My heart and my head are fully invested, and at the end of the day, I know my strengths and weaknesses—as all dentists should. My ethical code, for example, tells me not to perform procedures I don't enjoy, even if I am qualified to perform them. Root canals, for example, are something I don't like, so I won't do them. My patients often try to convince me to do their root canals—and I get it, they trust me—but I always refer them out for root canals.

In fact, dentists really shouldn't be touting themselves as jacks-of-all-trades. Most of us know what we do best and what we enjoy the most. As a patient, it is truly not in your best interest to beg your dentist, no matter how much you admire and respect him or her, to do work he or she is saying "No" to. For instance, I excel at implants, whereas most general dentists choose not to even perform the surgery, and I have done well over 1,000 of them. On the other hand, one of my colleagues is an expert in the field of TMD (Temporomandibular Joint Dysfunction). At one point in my career, embarrassed by my limited knowledge of the issue, I asked myself, "Should I go back to school to study TMD?" But no. Again, your dentist, like you, has a set of strengths and weaknesses and a set of likes and dislikes. I don't like root canals (they are painful, yes, but I also just don't enjoy doing them), and I know enough about TMD to know to send patients with it to my colleague, who is passionate about the disorder. By sending my root canal patients to the right person, I know they will get the best service from the person who is most in tune with this issue.

Do a little research before choosing a dentist. Talk to friends and coworkers, family, and even strangers in the street whose smiles floor you. A little knowledge goes a long way when searching for a dentist or a specialist of any kind. Trust your gut and remember, if your dentist suddenly tells you you need five cavities filled, a root canal or two, and possibly some veneers, raise your defense shields. If you sense something is "off," or if you hear your dentist explaining something he really seems to know nothing about, remember what is at stake. The number one complaint I hear from new patients is that they hate their teeth, and in many cases, this means that they hate what their former dentist has done to them—or may not have done for them.

> Trust your gut and remember, if your dentist suddenly tells you you need five cavities filled, a root canal or two, and possibly some veneers, raise your defense shields.

Yes, your life really is at stake when you are in the hands of a bad dentist, and we have certainly covered enough stories in this book. The truth is that most of us don't die from a rusty drill or a fluoride overdose, but many, many people have nearly died of embarrassment when a bad veneer has fallen off in their soup at their daughter's wedding. Many, many people have thrown thousands of dollars down that little dental sink drain they are told to spit into. We know that our teeth hold value beyond their function—we know that power, as well as physical and psychological wellbeing, comes from a healthy mouth. Know too, the two words you should always expect to hear from your dentist: "Let's talk."

CHAPTER 7

Is Your Dentist Slamming Too Many Patients in Order to Make a Living?

MANY OF US maintain the fantasy of the dentist taking off every afternoon to play golf or tennis, or jetting off to their second homes in Hawaii or Puerto Rico. We know that dentists all drive high-end European sports cars, and so do their spouses, right? They take vacation time whenever they darn well please, and they have an abundance of leisure time.

All this and more may have been true ... forty years ago. There were fewer practicing dentists, competition to get into dental schools wasn't as fierce, and student loans were unheard of. Nowadays, the truth for most of us is this: becoming a dentist does not make you an instant millionaire. It may be hard to believe, but your dentist may be broke. Most dentists, as I've said, struggle in their first few years out of dental school. Student loan debt is a serious issue for many. Graduating dental school owing $250,000 or more is normal, and people in their first year out of dental school can really only expect to make about $50,000.

When you note that our hourly rate is higher than that of other professions, please also remember that our overhead is through the roof. And not all freshly-minted dentists graduate with an ounce of business sense—so until they learn that too, life as a newbie dentist can be a challenge.

Yes, there are rich, Hollywood-type dentists who charge an arm and a leg because they can. And their patients pay top dollar not only because they can, but because for them it is all about status. "My friend spent $75K here last week. I'd like the same treatment." Some dentists can overcharge because they have a great reputation—their patients could do worse. But if we overlook these anomalies and focus on the typical dentist, what are we talking about in terms of income?

Even if a dentist owns her own practice and has 100 patients, she is hardly getting rich. Indeed, she may even have to wonder how she will make next month's rent. When you take this into consideration, you start to see how some dentists get to "find something … find anything wrong," so they can beef up their bottom lines. Fortunately, even in rough economic times, this kind of dentist is rare—word gets around, and practitioners who lack ethics are busted fairly quickly. Patients are educating themselves and sharing that knowledge via Facebook, Twitter, and other social media sites. Most dentists who unabashedly stick it to their patients are eventually ousted from the profession. A more common problem, however, is dentists who provide neglectful treatment.

Neglect in dentistry comes in many forms. At its extreme, of course, neglect can lead to death. These are cases that make national news and exacerbate the irrational fears about dentists many people already have. When news about bad dentists blows up, everyone becomes hyperaware—for a while. This book is meant to turn that fear and that hyperawareness into something else that lasts; this book is meant to educate people to educate themselves when it comes to their oral health, and to raise the bar all around.

> This book is meant to turn that fear and that hyperawareness into something else that lasts; this book is meant to educate people to educate themselves when it comes to their oral health, and to raise the bar all around.

Again, most neglect in dentistry does not lead to death, but the kind of neglect that leads to thousands upon thousands of dollars wasted can certainly kill a few dreams. You were planning to take the family to Florida for a week? You wanted to put a healthy down payment on a new car? You were finally about to pay off the last of your credit card debt in one celebratory swoop? Forget it— because your dentist was lazy and did not take an extra minute to ensure that all infection was cleared out before applying that cap, so in just a few weeks time you'll be needing additional surgeries and additional rounds of medications, which will cost you more than you bargained and budgeted for.

You do budget your money and your resources for healthcare. You expect your dental work to be done well and to be

> Look around, close your eyes, and take a deep breath—does the place feel right to you? Is the staff open and inviting and friendly, or are they sitting behind a closed window and gossiping loudly? Are the other patients waiting with you quietly enjoying magazines, or are they tapping their feet impatiently?

done right the first time. You also expect, as we touched on earlier, your dentist and his or her team to treat your personal schedule—your valuable time—with respect. I have stressed throughout this book the importance of trusting your gut in the waiting room. Look around, close your eyes, and take a deep breath—does the place feel right to you? Is the staff open and inviting and friendly, or are they sitting behind a closed window and gossiping loudly? Are the other patients waiting with you quietly enjoying magazines, or are they tapping their feet impatiently? Is your dentist running behind by ten minutes, or by a half hour? Is the waiting room jam-packed with dozens of impatient and overly anxious patients, or is there a nice, calm flow to the place?

Paying attention to waiting room details can tell you a lot. Your dentist may be cramming in patients for any number of reasons, none of them good. A jammed dentist is undoubtedly more prone to mistakes than a dentist who has trained his or her team to schedule patient visits well. Naturally, emergencies and last-minute issues happen in every medical field, but the best doctors and dentists begin their best treatment practices before they even see you. Would you want your mother to show up for an appointment on time and be made to wait twenty minutes in the waiting room and then an extra ten in the chair on top of that?

Do you want to be upsold every time you visit your dentist? Sure, maybe at the computer store you expect a little salesmanship—you go in for a new laptop and end up buying an external drive, two software programs you didn't even know you wanted, and a special three-year warranty plan that covers your new purchase against every possible danger under the sun. Upselling at your dentist, however, might mean a $600 cleaning is suggested when you only need the basic $150 treatment.

The average dentist's annual salary, depending on demographics, runs anywhere from $100,000 to $170,000. In dental offices across the country, millions of dollars change hands every year, and the best dentists run a smart and a tight ship when it comes to handling their patients' money. Dental office workers do not need degrees in finance, but they must be incredibly accurate and detail-oriented when it comes to insurance and billing matters. If someone starts missing or overcharging ten dollars here and there, dentists and patients lose. The fact is, most losses in billing errors come out of the dentist's pocket, which is why it behooves us to review our books at the end of every day.

Another issue patients should be aware of when it comes to insurance and billing is the need to go into their dentist's office

> Make sure, too, that your dentist or a member of the team is always amenable to discussing your insurance plan with you.

armed with a certain amount of knowledge. What is your premium? What is your copayment, if any? Are certain procedures deemed "purely cosmetic" and therefore not covered? Is there a yearly cap on your coverage? Insurance companies sometimes seem to specialize in the creation of imaginary worlds and extra fine print. Knowing the basics about your policy helps you and it helps your dentist. If your plan is unusually complicated, call your Human Resources department and ask someone to break it down into easier-to-digest numbers.

Make sure, too, that your dentist or a member of the team is always amenable to discussing your insurance plan with you. In my practice, it is standard operating procedure when we give a patient his or her treatment plan to also review with them what their insurance plan covers … or doesn't. In my office, we never do the work and then hand a patient the bill. Our patients are always informed about what they are up against. They are told that something unexpected could certainly come up, but here are our options if that becomes the case—and here is the bill you can expect, assuming all goes as planned.

We play fair. We aim to create awareness and smarts. No patient of mine would ever go in for heart surgery or knee replacement without knowing what it would cost them ahead of time, and they won't go in for three fillings without understanding the bill and what percentage of it they will pay.

The dental community, in general, is small and tight. We all suffered and survived the nightmare of dental school. We all, in general, keep one another in check. Many of us form lifelong partnerships and enjoy referring one another out so we always get to perform only the procedures we like the best. Most of us live by a code of ethics that encourages us to educate, respect, and care about one another, our patients, and our communities. In dentistry, there is no fear that we will become obsolete. No matter how good the science gets, the condition of the human mouth will always deteriorate. We dentists go into our profession because our passion is making that natural state of deterioration as pain free and as pleasant as possible. Most of us are not in this solely for the money. We are medical professionals who also value productivity, efficiency, and artistry—we run a business, which just happens to be a business of caring.

.

CHAPTER 8

Keeping an Open Mind:
Listening to Your Dentist

DREAMING OF LOSING your teeth is as common as dreaming of showing up to work naked or dreaming of flying. Dream analysis, for what it's worth, says that dreams about your teeth falling out mean you are feeling vulnerable in your waking life. These odd nightmares, in which you are powerless and suddenly all lip and gum, are said to be linked to concerns over losing a job, ending a relationship, or in the Freudian interpretation, sexual anxiety. Now of course not everyone remembers or interprets their dreams, but unfortunately, some of our worst dreams about our teeth do come true. You don't need a dentist to scare you about losing your teeth. We all know what happens when we play contact sports, or eat certain foods, or age—we have all caught glimpses of our grandparents' dentures floating in a cup.

In their waking lives, people lose teeth or veneers during vacations or important conferences. We go home after an exhilarating first date or an amazing job interview, only to look in the mirror and discover part of our lunch was stuck between our two front teeth. But dentists, too, have nightmares.

We have seen plenty. We have watched people open beer bottles and soda cans with their teeth. We have heard people chewing ice and those half-popped popcorn kernels at the movies. We have had patients come to us and explain that they had no other option but to super-glue part of their tooth back on: "I was at my cousin's wedding in rural Wyoming! What was I supposed to do?" Well, no one should ever put a caustic material in their mouth. Dentists have been asked to "clean up and reinsert" crowns that our patients have swallowed—yes, we have been asked to clean crowns that have made their way through our patients' digestive tracts and out the other end. We have seen the "emergency work" some of our patients have had done—out of desperation—while traveling abroad. We have seen everything, and sometimes what we see scares us.

Of course, we know how to fix things. This means, please, if you have chipped both your front teeth and have super-glued them back in place, do not hesitate one moment longer to get to your dentist. We will not lecture or shame you—our primary concern is to repair the damage and prevent worse things from happening.

• • •

We have talked about the small percentage of dentists out there who conduct themselves in a less-than-admirable or sometimes downright horrifying fashion. These dentists will try to shame you into getting work done that you do not need. Like the make-up counter salesgirl who tries to convince you that your face would look much younger if you purchased two more top-dollar products from their skin line, or the automobile sales team that wants you to believe everyone else is ordering all the upgrades, some dentists are in it to sell. Some dentists will play upon your worst fears and anxieties, subliminally or otherwise.

We have said more than once that if you are happy with your dentist, there is no need to start looking for problems— paranoia is no way to approach your health or your healthcare providers.

We have talked throughout this book about learning to trust your instincts. We have said more than once that if you are happy with your dentist, there is no need to start looking for problems—paranoia is no way to approach your health or your healthcare providers. You know the difference between the dentist who is offering you something and the dentist who is pushing it on you. In our office, for example, we hold up a shade guide to all our patients' teeth. We take baseline shade notes and enter them into our computer system in order to create a full health profile. If we detect significant changes in a patient's tooth coloration in an unusually short period of time, we'll dig deeper and ask that patient questions about his or her overall health and habits. When we do this quick shade analysis, roughly 30 percent of our patients ask, "What are you doing?" We explain that we are documenting the color of their teeth, so that five, ten, and twenty years from now, we can track any changes. Sometimes our patients raise an eyebrow and ask directly, "Are my teeth too yellow?" and then we will engage in dialogue.

How does a patient judge the color of his or her own teeth, or the quality of his or her own breath? We talk honestly with each patient in order to address these concerns, but in our practice, we consider it unethical to ever make a patient feel bad. Their teeth might be as yellow as summer sweet corn, but if the discoloration presents no threat to their health, and if the patient does not seem to be concerned, we do what we have to do during that visit and send them on their merry way—with a new soft toothbrush in hand.

It is hard to put a precise dollar amount on what any given dental treatment should cost because this number fluctuates so much, depending on geography. East and West Coast dentists, in general, are more expensive than their Midwest counterparts. When it comes to determining whether your dentist's pricing scale is fair, doing a bit of research and talking to your friends will help. Ask your friends and colleagues about their dentists. You'd be surprised, given the power of today's social media and networking tools, how often you might find yourself just one degree removed from someone who actually works in a dental office. Find a way to contact that person and ask questions. Links and resources to finding your best fit are more numerous and accessible than ever.

Putting a precise dollar amount on a healthy mouth is impossible. Ask any of your friends or family members what they would pay for a beautiful smile—chances are they won't even be able to come up with a number. Defining what a healthy mouth is also presents a challenge. In some parts of the country, a missing tooth is no big deal. Plenty of people wander through their days with halitosis and find chewing gum a perfectly acceptable solution. "I've got a little bit of decay on a tooth nobody can even see?" some people might say, "So what!" But most of us would pay anything for a clean, fresh, pain-free, beautiful healthy mouth. The truth is, nothing is more rewarding to your dentist than to see you every six months and to be able to say, "Great job taking care of your oral health!"

CHAPTER 9

How to Choose a Dentist
Who Will Take Great Care of You

YOUR SMILE IS one of your greatest assets, and you must protect it. Again, you are not a shark—if you want to keep your teeth, you have to brush them. If you want fresh breath and healthy gums, use the proper toothbrush and floss and

> Your smile is one of your greatest assets, and you must protect it.

stay hydrated. Visit your dentist regularly, and stay aware of your own health and body. Talk to your dentist and dental assistant, and ask questions whenever you are unsure. Remember, most dentists got into their profession because of a deep-seated passion for taking care of people—there is no need to dread visiting your dentist.

If in reading through this book, you have come to the happy conclusion that you have the best dentist for you—congratulations! My goal was not to put all patients on high alert. I trust you to trust your instinct, and if you've got it good, stay where you are. If, on the other hand, this book hit a nerve, so to speak, congratulations to you, too. Now you have the knowledge you need; now you know it's probably time either to begin asking questions or to begin to shop around for a new dentist.

Good dentists want you to arrive at ease—they are not rushed or insecure, and therefore are not bothered when you ask what you can do to take better care of yourself. The more you are able to attend to your oral health daily at home, the happier good dentists are. When you have pain, we prefer you don't suffer for days, hoping it will recede on its own; we want you to visit us right away. When you are in a tight financial space, we want you to know that money you put off spending now will likely result in greater costs later, and that we offer options—so visit us.

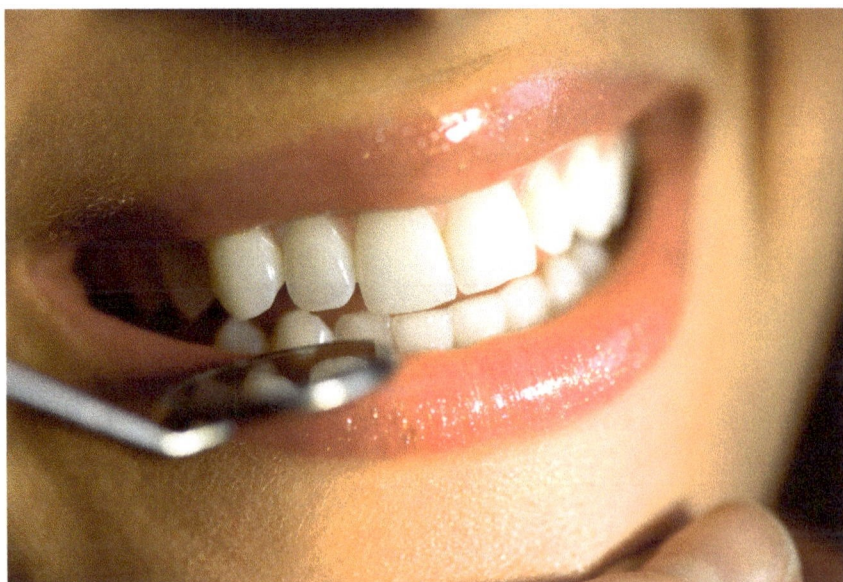

I realize that people may assume my goal in writing this book is to drum up more business for my office—that is untrue.

What I do want to offer, though, is a link to my website, www.TheTroothInDentistry.com, where you can click on the tab *Find a Great Dentist*. I have begun a movement on the East Coast, with the intent to build a national list of honest and ethical dentists, ordered by ZIP code. If you have exhausted recommendations from all your family and friends, or have moved to a new city, or are just unsure of where to find a great dentist, this resource is for you. Our link is constantly updated, with new *Great Dentists* added on a regular basis. If you cannot locate a *Great Dentist* in your area, you can e-mail us via another link provided on the site, and we will do our best to serve you.

Being in this profession for so long means I have networked with dentists from all over the country and have gotten to know who does what best—from the West Coast to the East Coast. Type your ZIP code into the *Great Dentists Movement Find a Great Dentist Near Me* system, and you will find a list of dentists in your area whom I either know personally or who have developed unparalleled reputations, or who may be new to the field but exhibit stellar credentials and provide top-notch references.

Besides this website, I have included a checklist below, of questions and ideas for your next dentist visit, that will help.

Keep in mind these are not set in stone—you don't have to do all, or any of these things, or you can expand upon what I suggest. My list may or may not fit the needs of one particular person. Use it if you need a little extra help in making a decision regarding a dentist.

Your Checklist:
- How long will you spend with me on the first visit?
- Is it okay for me to ask questions?
- How can I be a better patient, or even your best patient?
- Do you generally run on time for appointments?
- If I were unhappy with a service, how would you handle it?
- What is your favorite aspect of dentistry?
- What is your least favorite aspect of dentistry?
- Do you feel I am a good fit as a patient in your practice?

Remember we all share the freedom of choice. You can choose to ask your dentist and his or her staff questions if you want.

Other ideas:
- Visit the office for a walk through.
- Have a private five-minute talk with at least two office employees.
- Visit your State Dental Board's website. Review the dentist to see if any action has been taken against him or her. Keep in mind that while some of the content you read online may be very helpful, some may be misleading. If you find something disturbing, take the time to look into it further. You

may also want to give the dentist a chance to explain the situation by asking him about it personally in a non-threatening way.

- Ask some local people if they would recommend that dental office.
- See what type of organizations the dentist belongs to.

Beware of:
- Patients who talk badly about the dentist, but offer no specifics to prove their complaints or claims.
- Online reviews. Most online reviews are written when people are soured about one particular event (usually involving money). Not all online reviews tell the whole story about a particular dentist's character and practice.
- An office where blood and contamination are clearly visible.
- A dentist who is extremely rude or verbally abusive toward either patients or employees.

I leave you with this important closing thought – your health is the number one thing you have to attend to throughout your lives. Excellent oral health practices, in particular, must be started early in life—while you may be able to "ignore" your arteries in your youth, you cannot go until you are fifty-five without brushing your teeth. Now more than ever, many of us have become

> Together, you and your dentist can work to ensure that you enter and exit that dental chair smiling every single time.

more vigilant about all aspects of how we take care of ourselves. We order fruits and vegetables from our local community farms or shop at the farmers' market. We run, swim, or walk to maintain a decent level of fitness. We also attend to the cosmetic—we color our hair or whiten our teeth, and so on. The point is, you may do all the right things for your heart, muscles, bones, and skin, but if you neglect your oral health, the quality of your life will suffer.

Your mouth requires great care, and you deserve a great dentist. Together, you and your dentist can work to ensure that you enter and exit that dental chair smiling every single time.

www.ingramcontent.com/pod-product-compliance
Lightning Source LLC
Chambersburg PA
CBHW060318310326
41914CB00101B/1982/J